KIDNEY STONES

DIET

FOR NOVICES

Enriched Recipes, Foods, Meal Plan & Procedures For Kidney Health, Recovery, Healing, Wellness, Nourishment, Optimal Well-Being And More

DR. MATEO GABRIEL

DISCLAIMER

The information in this book is only meant to be used for general reading. In any way, the author and publisher do not promise or represent that the information in this work is full, correct, reliable, appropriate, or available. This includes any warranties that are expressed or implied. Because of this, you should only rely on this material at your own risk.

This book is not meant to replace professional help. If you have any questions about a subject, you should always get help from a qualified expert. The author and distributor of this book are not responsible for how the information in it is used or abused.

The author's thoughts and feelings are shown in this book. They do not necessarily represent the official policy or stance of any other person, group, employer, or business.

Any third-party material that you can get to through this book is not endorsed or backed by the author or publisher.

The information in this book is correct at the time it was published, after all possible checks. However, the author and distributor are not responsible for any loss, damage, or inconvenience that may be caused by mistakes or omissions.

TABLE OF CONTENTS

CHAPTER ONE

INTRODUCTION TO KIDNEY STONES DIET

Nephrolithiasis, the medical term for kidney stones, is the term used to describe solid deposits in the kidneys caused by compounds found in the urine. These stones range in size from small particles to massive constructions the size of golf balls. Kidney stones can cause excruciating pain and agony and interfere with the urinary system's ability to operate normally. It is essential to comprehend kidney stone kinds, causes, and symptoms to effectively avoid and treat kidney stones.

MEANING AND CATEGORIES

There are various forms of kidney stones, and each is distinguished by the particular materials that comprise the stone. Calcium stones, which are made of calcium phosphate or calcium oxalate, are the most prevalent kind. Uric acid stones, cystine stones, and struvite stones are among more forms. The treatment and preventative techniques for a stone are influenced by its makeup.

REASONS AND DANGER FACTORS

Kidney stones can develop for a variety of reasons. One of the main causes is dehydration because concentrated urine can encourage the crystallization of minerals. Dietary elements may also be involved, such as consuming an excessive amount of foods high in oxalate or animal proteins. Kidney stone production may be more likely in people with specific medical problems, such as metabolic abnormalities and urinary tract infections. The risk factors for this ailment can also include obesity, a family history of kidney stones, and certain drugs.

TYPICAL SYMPTOMS

Kidney stones can cause excruciating discomfort in the back or side, among other symptoms. Renal colic is the name for this pain, which can also spread to the groin and lower abdomen. People may have a constant urge to urinate in addition to experiencing pain when urinating. Another typical sign of kidney stones is hematuria or blood in the urine. These symptoms may be accompanied by nausea, vomiting, and fever, which could be signs of infection or other problems.

Recognizing these typical symptoms is necessary for an early diagnosis and course of treatment. Early identification reduces the risk of consequences including kidney damage and urinary tract infections and enables more effective care of kidney stones.

CHAPTER TWO

HOW URINARY STONES DEVELOP

FORMATION METHOD

Minerals in the urine crystallize to form kidney stones, also known as renal calculi, in a convoluted process. The main constituents of kidney stones are phosphate, calcium, and oxalate, which can precipitate as solid particles when their concentration in the urine rises too high. The supersaturation of urine, in which the concentration of these minerals is above the solubility limit, is the first stage in the production of stones.

Consequently, crystals start to precipitate and gather, creating the core of the stone.

These crystal formations may then enlarge and transform into kidney stones. The pH of the urine, the presence of certain chemicals that either hinder or promote crystal formation, and the total volume of urine are some of the elements that affect the growth and maturation of stones. In addition, the absence of adequate inhibitors in the urine may allow crystals to aggregate and form larger, more solid stones.

FACTORS AFFECTING THE FORMATION OF STONE

Kidney stone development is a complex process that is influenced by multiple factors. Dehydration plays a major role since less fluid intake causes concentrated urine, which raises the possibility of crystal formation. Dietary variables are also important; eating a lot of foods high in oxalate, such as chocolate, almonds, and beets, can lead to the production of stones. Moreover, consuming too much salt—especially sodium—can raise the excretion of calcium in the urine, which encourages the development of calcium-based stones.

Another factor that may raise a person's risk of kidney stones is genetic predisposition. Those who have a family history of stone formation may be predisposed to specific genetic features that impact how their systems metabolize and eliminate minerals. Metabolic problems like hyperparathyroidism or certain kidney disorders can also cause the body's normal mineral balance to be upset, which can lead to the formation of stones.

DIAGNOSTIC TECHNIQUES

A combination of imaging techniques, laboratory testing, and clinical assessment is usually used to diagnose kidney stones. A thorough medical history is frequently part of the initial evaluation to determine the symptoms and risk factors related to stone formation. A routine diagnostic procedure called a urinalysis can detect blood, crystals, or unusually high concentrations of specific chemicals in the urine, which can provide important information about the possibility of kidney stones.

Finding the size and position of the stones as well as validating the diagnosis depend heavily on imaging studies. Kidney stones are extremely visible on non-contrast computed tomography (CT) images because of their high density. Additionally, ultrasound imaging may be utilized, especially in situations like pregnancy when CT scans are not advised.

In certain cases, post-passage laboratory study of the stone's composition or surgical removal might yield important details about the type of stone and help determine the best course of treatment. Blood tests may also be performed to evaluate kidney function and find any underlying metabolic problems that could be causing stones. When these diagnostic tests are used comprehensively, medical professionals can create customized treatment strategies for patients with kidney stones.

CHAPTER THREE
KIDNEY STONE TYPES
OXALATE STONES OF CALCIUM

Crystalline deposits known as kidney stones develop in the kidneys as a result of specific compounds in the urine condensing. Calcium oxalate kidney stones are the most prevalent kind of kidney stone. These stones occur when solid crystals of calcium and oxalate mix in the urine. Managing calcium oxalate stones require a low-sodium lifestyle. Sodium can enhance the excretion of calcium in the urine, resulting in raised levels and a heightened risk of stone formation. As a result, low-sodium diets are frequently recommended for people who have a history of calcium oxalate stones to reduce their risk.

STONES WITH URIC ACID

On the other side, uric acid crystallization in the urine causes uric acid stones. It is also advantageous to lead a low-sodium lifestyle to avoid uric acid stones. Because salt can affect how much uric acid is excreted, cutting back on sodium intake helps to maintain a more ideal balance and reduces the risk of developing stones. Furthermore, since increased uric acid levels are a typical precursor to both gout and uric acid stones, a low-sodium diet is generally advised for those who are prone to gout.

STONES OF STRUVITE

Although rare, struvite stones can be extremely dangerous to one's health. The main elements of these stones are phosphate, ammonium, and magnesium. Because certain bacteria can create chemicals that encourage the production of struvite crystals, they frequently arise from urinary tract infections. Adopting a low-sodium lifestyle does not directly prevent struvite stones from occurring.

On the other hand, while treating urinary tract infections early on might help prevent stones, it is imperative to address the underlying reasons.

KIDNEY STONES

Rarely, do cystine stones develop from a genetic condition that leads the kidneys to eliminate too much of certain amino acids, including cystine. Although avoiding salt may not be the major strategy for preventing kidney stones, keeping the kidneys healthy overall is crucial. Combining a healthy diet with adequate fluid consumption can help lower the incidence of kidney stones by reducing the amount of cystine in the urine.

Furthermore, as cystinuria may affect the excretion of specific amino acids, controlling salt intake is essential for those who have the condition.

A low-sodium diet is a major factor in preventing the development of different kinds of kidney stones. Reducing sodium intake aids in keeping the excretion of uric acid and calcium in balance, which is beneficial for both uric acid and calcium oxalate stones. Reducing salt may not have a direct effect on struvite and cystine stones, but a well-balanced diet and adequate hydration are crucial for preserving kidney function in general and preventing these less prevalent forms of kidney stones.

Kidney stone sufferers should collaborate closely with medical professionals to create customized food programs that target their unique risk factors and support healthy kidney function.

CHAPTER FOUR

DIET'S PART IN PREVENTING KIDNEY STONES

The function that nutrition plays in the development and recurrence of kidney stones makes it impossible to overestimate the significance of diet in kidney stone prevention. When certain minerals, such as calcium, oxalate, and phosphorus, concentrate in the urine, solid deposits known as kidney stones can develop in the kidneys. A focused and well-balanced diet can significantly lower a person's chance of acquiring kidney stones.

DIETARY RECOMMENDATIONS TO AVOID KIDNEY STONES

The significance of controlling the consumption of particular minerals and chemicals is emphasized in dietary guidelines for the prevention of stones. Limiting the consumption of foods high in oxalate is important because too much oxalate can lead to the development of calcium oxalate stones, which are the most frequent kinds of kidney stones. Edibles high in oxalate include chocolate, almonds, beets, and several leafy greens. Reducing salt intake is also crucial since high sodium can cause increased excretion of calcium in the urine, which can exacerbate the formation of stones.

WATER BALANCE AND KIDNEY STONES

Kidney stone prevention relies heavily on hydration, and sustaining a sufficient water intake is essential to this strategy. Maintaining adequate hydration lowers the concentration of minerals and other chemicals in the urine, which lessens the risk of stones forming. It is generally recommended that people consume at least 8 glasses of water a day, while exact amounts may differ depending on variables like weather, level of physical activity, and general health.

IMPORTANCE OF CONSUMING ENOUGH WATER

It is impossible to exaggerate the importance of drinking enough water when trying to prevent kidney stones. As a natural solvent, water keeps salts and minerals from crystallizing and producing kidney stones. Additionally, maintaining adequate hydration encourages normal urine flow, which aids in clearing the urinary tract of any materials that may form stones. One easy yet effective strategy that people can use to reduce their risk of kidney stones is to drink enough water.

FLUID TYPES AND THEIR EFFECTS

Kidney stone prevention is impacted by fluids in several ways. Although water is the primary and most advised fluid for hydration, other drinks can also be included in the total amount of fluid consumed. Because citrate helps prevent some forms of kidney stones from forming, citrus liquids like lemonade have been demonstrated to be useful. Drinks heavy in sugar or caffeine should be consumed with caution, though, as this can hurt kidney function. Finding the right balance between adding excess amounts of chemicals that may promote the production of stones and fluids that maintain hydration is crucial.

A low-sodium lifestyle is a complex strategy to lower the incidence of kidney stones. It should be accompanied by adherence to dietary guidelines for stone prevention and an emphasis on proper hydration. People can actively manage their health and help prevent kidney stones by making educated decisions about what they eat and drink. This promotes overall kidney health and well-being.

CHAPTER FIVE

NUTRITIONAL ASPECTS OF KIDNEY STONE DEVELOPMENT

RICH IN OXALATE FOODS

Given that oxalate is a naturally occurring substance in a wide variety of plant-based diets, oxalate-rich foods are important in the development of kidney stones. Overconsumption of oxalate can cause it to bind with calcium in the urine, creating crystals that can eventually cause kidney stones. Foods high in oxalates include chocolate, almonds, spinach, and beets. It's common advice for people who are prone to kidney stones to limit their consumption of certain foods to lower their chance of developing stones. It's crucial to remember, though, that not everyone who eats foods high in oxalate will have kidney stones because stone production is also influenced by other variables like heredity and general health.

INGESTION OF CALCIUM

Consuming calcium is another important component when it comes to the development of kidney stones. Even though it may seem paradoxical, consuming enough calcium in your diet can help prevent kidney stones. In the digestive tract, calcium binds to oxalate to minimize the quantity that reaches the kidneys and the chance of crystal formation. Maintaining a healthy calcium intake from dietary sources such as dairy products, leafy greens, and fortified meals is crucial for people who are at risk of kidney stones. Achieving the ideal balance is crucial since overdoing calcium supplements without adequate water can exacerbate the development of stones.

SALT AND SODIUM INTAKE

Consumption of salt and sodium is also a major factor in the development of kidney stones, especially those made of calcium oxalate. Increased calcium output through the urine due to a high sodium diet can raise the concentration of calcium in the kidneys and encourage the production of stones. A high-sodium diet can also cause dehydration, which lowers urine volume and concentration and speeds up the process of minerals crystallizing in the kidneys. For those who are prone to kidney stones, a low-sodium lifestyle is advised to reduce these risks. To support general kidney health, this means minimizing the use of table salt, avoiding high-sodium processed and packaged foods, and embracing fresh, natural foods.

A thorough strategy for preventing kidney stones entails giving considerable thought to dietary decisions about sodium, calcium, and oxalate-rich foods. For those who are at risk of kidney stones, it is essential to maintain proper hydration and strike a balance between these elements. While some dietary changes may be helpful, it's crucial to speak with medical professionals so that suggestions can be customized to address unique risk factors and medical problems.

RECOGNIZING PH BALANCE

When discussing the development of kidney stones, an understanding of pH balance is essential. The term pH level describes how acidic or basic a substance is, and in the case of the human body, it is crucial for preserving homeostasis. The kidneys are in charge of controlling the pH of the body by eliminating surplus acids or bases. However, kidney stones can develop as a result of a pH imbalance. Crystals that can grow in an environment that is either too acidic or too alkaline are often the building blocks of kidney stones.

ALKALINE AND ACIDIC FOODS

Acidic foods or alkaline are important factors in determining the pH levels of the body. The consumption of acidic foods, such as various meats, dairy products, and cereals, can cause the body to produce more acid. Conversely, meals high in alkalis, such as fruits, vegetables, and legumes, can counteract the effects of acids. Maintaining a healthy balance between these acidic and alkaline meals is crucial to avoiding the development of kidney stones. The objective is to keep the body's environment somewhat alkaline because too acidic conditions can encourage the crystallization of minerals, which can result in kidney stones.

PH BALANCING TO AVOID STONES

Maintaining a pH balance to prevent stones requires eating a diet high in alkaline-forming foods and low in acid-forming ones. Citrate-rich foods, such as oranges and lemons, have been demonstrated to prevent the development of several kinds of kidney stones. Furthermore, consuming more alkalizing foods like spinach, kale, and broccoli can help maintain a more balanced pH.

It's important to remember that maintaining pH balance and preventing kidney stones both depend heavily on staying hydrated. Drinking enough water helps dilute chemicals in the urine, which reduces the likelihood of crystals forming. People who are predisposed to kidney stones should drink enough water since concentrated urine promotes the growth of crystals.

Knowledge of pH balance is essential to understanding kidney stone formation dynamics.

CHAPTER SIX

PLANS FOR KIDNEY STONE DIETS

GENERAL DIETARY ADVICE

Managing and preventing kidney stones are greatly aided by following a kidney stone diet plan. Adopting a dietary strategy that lowers the likelihood of specific minerals crystallizing and creating kidney stones is the main goal. One of the main suggestions is to drink more fluids, especially water, to ensure enough hydration and to dilute chemicals that may cause stones to form.

People on a kidney stone diet should concentrate on eating a range of nutrient-rich meals in addition to drinking enough water. Essential vitamins and minerals can be obtained via a balanced diet that consists of a variety of fruits, vegetables, whole grains, and lean proteins without overdoing the body with ingredients that can cause stones. Reducing the consumption of specific foods that are high in oxalates, such as chocolate, almonds, tea, and beets, is also often advised because excessive oxalate can lead to the development of calcium oxalate stones.

RECOMMENDED DAILY ALLOWANCES

Creating a kidney stone diet plan that works requires understanding and following recommended daily allowances (RDAs). RDAs offer recommendations for the consumption of vital nutrients, assisting people in meeting their dietary requirements without going overboard and possibly causing health problems like kidney stones. For example, it's important to keep your calcium consumption within reasonable limits because too much or too little calcium might cause stones.

Consumption of sodium is another important consideration because elevated sodium levels can cause increased excretion of calcium in the urine, which may aid in the development of calcium-containing stones. In keeping with general health recommendations for blood pressure management and cardiovascular health, monitoring and regulating sodium consumption is recommended. Maintaining equilibrium in the consumption of different nutrients, such as sodium, calcium, and oxalates, is crucial in averting the recurrence of kidney stones.

PORTION CONTROL AND BALANCED MEALS

Keeping a healthy weight and controlling caloric intake are key goals of kidney stone diet plans. Portion management is a key component of these plans. Limiting portion sizes can improve general health and lower the chance of obesity, which is associated with a higher chance of kidney stones developing. Furthermore, consuming food in moderation throughout the day and including balanced meals will help control insulin swings and blood sugar levels, improving metabolic health.

A range of micronutrients from various food sources are combined with a mix of macronutrients, such as proteins, fats, and carbs, to create balanced meals. By guaranteeing that the body gets a wide range of vital nutrients, this balance promotes general health and helps prevent kidney stones from forming. Portion control and a focus on well-balanced meals together provide a sustainable dietary approach that supports kidney stone prevention while also promoting general well-being.

INCLUDING VEGETABLES AND FRUITS

Kidney stones are solid deposits that can form in the kidneys from minerals and salts. A kidney stone diet plan is essential for controlling and preventing kidney stones. An essential component of such a regimen is including a range of fruits and vegetables in the diet. These foods help support overall kidney health since they are high in fiber, antioxidants, and vital nutrients. In addition, fruits and vegetables usually include a lot of water, which helps you stay hydrated and prevents the concentration of minerals that might cause stones to form.

REDUCED-OXALATE CHOICES

It's critical to consider the oxalate concentration of specific foods when following a kidney stone diet. Many plant-based meals contain oxalates, which are substances that are known to play a role in the development of kidney stones made of calcium oxalate. Including low-oxalate choices becomes crucial for people who are prone to oxalate-based stones. This entails limiting the consumption of foods high in oxalates, such as spinach, beets, and almonds, and selecting fruits and vegetables that are lower in oxalates, such as berries, apples, cabbage, and cauliflower.

DECISIONS THAT GENERATE AN ALKALINE

A kidney stone diet plan should also encourage the consumption of alkaline-forming foods. Foods with an alkaline effect on the body can aid in balancing the acidic environments that could be linked to kidney stone development. Fruits and vegetables are important in this regard; alkaline-forming foods include citrus fruits, melons, and leafy greens. These options supply vital vitamins and minerals that assist kidney function in addition to helping to maintain the pH balance of the body overall.

A diet plan for kidney stones that emphasizes the consumption of fruits and vegetables is a comprehensive strategy for maintaining kidney health. An all-encompassing dietary approach includes combining alkaline-forming options with low-oxalate alternatives to balance the oxalate concentration. In addition, keeping a diet full of vital minerals and drinking enough water supports healthy kidney function and lowers the chance of kidney stones. Before implementing a diet plan, people should speak with a medical expert or a qualified dietitian to discuss their needs and medical history.

CHAPTER SEVEN

DIETARY STRATEGIES FOR PARTICULAR STONE TYPES

CALCIUM OXALATE STONE DIET

Limiting oxalate intake is the main nutritional strategy for people who are at risk of developing calcium oxalate stones. Foods high in oxalate, like chocolate, almonds, beets, and other vegetables, should be eaten in moderation. It is advised to consume enough calcium since it can bind to oxalates in the intestines and stop them from being absorbed and causing stones to develop. Since more fluids help dilute the concentration of calcium and oxalate in the urine, staying hydrated is essential for preventing calcium oxalate stones.

Dietary changes to reduce urinary acidity and purine-rich meals are necessary to manage the production of uric acid stones. It is recommended that people reduce their intake of shellfish, organ meats, and vegetables high in purines. It's critical to stay well-hydrated since it dissolves uric acid crystals and keeps them from clumping together to form stones. Under medical supervision, alkalinizing medicines like potassium citrate may be suggested to increase urine pH and lower the risk of uric acid stone formation.

Dietary precautions should be taken in addition to treating the underlying infection to avoid the formation of struvite stones, which are frequently caused by urinary tract infections. Struvite stone development may be avoided by acidifying the urine with a diet low in alkaline foods, such as some fruits and vegetables. Furthermore, to reduce the chance of a recurrence of stone disease, those with a history of struvite stones should exercise caution when consuming foods high in phosphorus, such as dairy products.

CYSTINE STONE DIET

A genetic disease inhibiting the renal reabsorption of the amino acid cystine is the cause of cystine stones. Keeping a low-cystine diet, which includes limiting the consumption of high-cystine foods such as red meat, eggs, and dairy products, is essential to managing the formation of cystine stones. Drinking enough water is essential to reducing the concentration of cystine in the urine and diluting it, which prevents the formation of stones. To further reduce the levels of cystine in the urine, doctors may further prescribe medications like tiopronin.

Low-Sodium Lifestyle: To prevent different kinds of kidney stones, it's imperative to adopt a low-sodium lifestyle. Increased excretion of calcium in the urine due to a high-sodium diet can exacerbate the development of calcium-based stones.

CHAPTER EIGHT

WAY OF LIFE AND ADDITIONAL FACTORS

PHYSICAL ACTIVITY AND WEIGHT MANAGEMENT

Achieving and maintaining a healthy weight through appropriate weight management is essential to avoiding the development of kidney stones. Kidney stones are one kind of stone that can develop as a result of being overweight. Conditions like hyperoxaluria and hypercalciuria, which raise the risk of stone formation, are frequently linked to obesity. In addition to helping to manage weight, a healthy diet high in fruits, vegetables, and whole grains together with regular exercise can help lower the risk of stone formation.

Engaging in physical exercise is a crucial part of maintaining a healthy lifestyle and may help avoid the formation of stones. Frequent exercise helps maintain ideal body weight and enhances general well-being. Furthermore, by improving bone health and lowering the risk of diseases like osteoporosis, physical activity can help prevent kidney stones. Exercises involving weight bearing, in particular, can improve bone density and reduce the amount of calcium released into the urine, hence reducing the chance of developing calcium-based stones.

EFFECT ON FORMATION OF STONES

Numerous factors, such as nutrition, hydration, and genetic susceptibility, affect the production of stones. A sedentary lifestyle and unhealthful eating habits are two lifestyle choices that can raise the risk of stone formation. Dehydration is a prevalent component in the creation of stones because concentrated urine creates a crystal-forming environment. Together with a healthy diet and regular exercise, drinking enough water can help dilute urine and lower the concentration of minerals that cause stones to develop.

EXERCISE SUGGESTIONS

Regular physical exercise is essential for maintaining general health and well-being and can play a major role in preventing the formation of stones. A minimum of 150 minutes of moderate-intensity aerobic exercise per week is advised by the American College of Sports Medicine, along with two or more days of muscle-strengthening activities. Exercises that promote weight management, such as strength and cardio training, also improve bone health and lower the risk of disorders linked to the development of stones.

CHAPTER NINE

MEDICATIONS AND SUPPLEMENTS

SUPPLEMENTS OF VITAMINS AND MINERALS

Supplements containing specific vitamins and minerals may help avoid stones. For example, since vitamin B6 aids in the body's breakdown of oxalate, increasing vitamin B6 consumption may help lower the chance of oxalate stone development. Sufficient consumption of vitamin D can improve bone health and potentially lower the risk of calcium-based stones by facilitating the absorption and utilization of calcium. However, before adding supplements to one's regimen, it is imperative to speak with a healthcare provider because taking too much of them can have negative effects.

DRUGS FOR THE PREVENTION OF STONES

Healthcare professionals may occasionally recommend medicine to stop kidney stones from coming again. For example, thiazide diuretics can be used to lessen the risk of calcium-based stone formation by decreasing the excretion of calcium in the urine. For people who are prone to uric acid stones, allopurinol may be administered to lower uric acid levels. Medication containing citrate can raise urine citrate levels, which prevents some kinds of stones from forming. To evaluate the efficacy and safety of these drugs, patients must carefully adhere to their healthcare provider's instructions and receive routine monitoring.

ORGANIZING MEALS AND RECIPES

Planning your meals is essential to keeping up a balanced and healthful lifestyle. It entails giving careful thought to dietary constraints, individual preferences, and nutritional needs. Making example meal plans is a useful strategy for meal planning. These meal plans provide a balanced and nutrient-rich diet in addition to streamlining the preparation procedure. A well-designed sample meal plan considers the distribution of macronutrients, the number of calories consumed each day, and the inclusion of multiple food groups.

Specialized meal planning is crucial when it comes to preserving renal health. Meal plans that are healthy for the kidneys emphasize limiting certain nutrients, such as potassium, salt, and phosphorus, which might affect kidney function. It is usually beneficial for people with renal problems to speak with a medical practitioner or a qualified dietitian to customize meal plans to meet their requirements.

RECIPES SUITABLE FOR KIDNEYS

Recipes that are suitable for kidneys are essential for helping those who have kidney problems. These dishes are meant to be savory and filling but low in phosphorus, potassium, and salt. Varietal fruits and vegetables, lean meats, and minimal dairy are common components of kidney-friendly dishes. These dishes frequently highlight cooking techniques that preserve nutrients without using excessive quantities of salt or other additions.

Developing a recipe book for kidney-friendly dishes enables people with renal issues to eat a good and varied diet without sacrificing their health. A crucial component of effective meal planning for kidney health is modifying recipes to meet specific needs and preferences, which can differ from person to person.

A holistic approach to well-being takes into accounts not only food requirements but also lifestyle elements including physical activity, hydration, and stress management. An all-around healthy lifestyle includes frequent exercise, drinking enough water, and using stress-reduction strategies.

In the end, finding kidney-friendly dishes and mastering the art of meal planning are dynamic endeavors that demand constant care and adjustment. Through the adoption of a deliberate and personalized lifestyle approach, people can develop behaviors that support not only kidney health but also general well-being and lifespan.